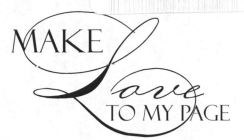

MAKE *Love* TO MY PAGE

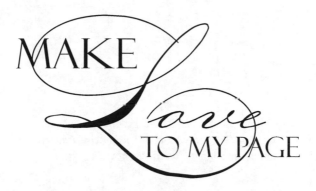

MAKE Love TO MY PAGE

A book of erotic love poems

V. E. SWANIGAN

authorHOUSE®

AuthorHouse™ LLC
1663 Liberty Drive
Bloomington, IN 47403
www.authorhouse.com
Phone: 1-800-839-8640

Published by AuthorHouse 01/28/2014

ISBN: 978-1-4918-5228-6 (sc)
ISBN: 978-1-4918-5223-1 (e)

Library of Congress Control Number: 2014900803

Table of Contents

Speechless

I am never speechless

But you leave me breathless

I feel my words tripping over my tongue

Cause I do not want to say the words wrong

I am tied up in knots

Cause you hit all the right spots

My toes are curling up like a curling iron burned it up

I can't think straight so my thoughts shut up

My heart is lost for words

So my sounds are not heard

You breathe life into me to a point I am mute

This amount of love my brain can't compute

I am normally calculated in every way

Savvy articulated in every word I say

But near you I stutter and fumble

It's like watching Michael Jordan double dribble

I get paid to speak up, out loud, and to let the world know

But with you my heart races

My mouth collapses

And all I want is for time to stand still or just move slow

And maybe in between the seconds I can get the chance to let you know

That my unconditional love is something that shall continue to grow

V. E. Swanigan

From First Sight

Looking across the room for a comfortable place

My vision is halted by the glare of your face

It was like we both fell into a trance

And all it took was one quick glance

Stunned by beauty

Sudden breaths of ecstasy

Pulled into an easy conversation

Found myself walking in your direction

Reminding myself every second to take it slow

Not sure how far this impulsive attraction will go

The distance between us extended by money and time

But not stopping you from running through my mind

Because I enjoy hearing you talk

And watching the way you walk

Standing next to you for some reason feels right

Peace comes as we lay throughout the night

Contemplating what was and what shall be

Wondering about the next time I can have thee

V. E. Swanigan

You're Simple

There is something about you that simply amazes

Makes me believe you were blessed by God's graces

You speak with authority in your diction

And passion in your conviction

While showing pure compassion in your affection

There is something about you that makes me melt inside

You are so warm that I never want to go outside

And you make me sing I'll stand by your side

While submitting to you my mind and body to guide

You are simple in your delivery

Your love takes over me

Slow kisses never missing a spot

A single pleasure that makes me hot

Never too complex or complicated

In your truth that is how we made it

V. E. Swanigan

I Like It Black

Like Folgers in the morning you're the excitement that starts my day

Raising my temperature, making me smile and sending me on my way

I like you hot and steamy fresh out the pot

You brew my dreams and stain my thought

I love to lick the rim of your cup

Give it to me straight up

No Styrofoam or plastic; I need the real thing porcelain hard and strong

I could drink you all day and night long

An exotic twist of sweet Verona no milk no sugar

I prefer it all black hell go figure

It feels better on my tongue and it keeps me warm

So cozy you make me feel like I shall never see harm

They say the blacker the berry the sweeter the juice

Well the blacker the bean the more I go through the roof

You're simply smooth

I love the way you make me move

I need you to awaken me and sooth my soul

Something about you makes me lose control

Right at the end I'll add a little cream

Drink to the last drop cause you make me steam

The perfect stimulus to arouse my sensation

V. E. Swanigan

You have me so relaxed; released my tension

You cleanse and filter out the dreariness of my day

You even keep me from getting in my own way

You're the best part of waking up

A rich pure taste that fills me up

It's a tantalizing classic dark roast

So damn good I make a toast

Nothing in robust flavor do you lack

So, Baby, give it to me black

Passions Tone

Passions tone

Making love on the phone

It rings and I know it's you ready to make my body moan

The whisper of your voice

The melody of your conversation

Adding to the personal pleasure

My body must rejoice

Escalating to the rhythm

Following your every command

My body complies with only your demand

Craving your touch

But pleased by longing for such

Twisting and turning in my bed

Barely able to breathe as my legs spread

Oh right there say it again

The sounds of you overwhelm me until orgasm

My body relaxes in a passionate chill

Your resonating voice gives me a thrill

And in an instant BEEP Oh damn call waiting

I guess for the next time I'll be anticipating

V. E. Swanigan

Thinking About You

When I think about you

My mind imagines the length of your spine

I recall my fingers tracing your smile line

I recognize your voice in my heart beat

It still makes me tingle down to my feet

I just want to be close to you

If only for a second of your time

I would love to press rewind

When I think about you

I remember the pressure from your lips

And the way your hands pressed on my hips

I still know the tickle of the hairs from your chin

Wrestled down by your love, I enjoyed feeling you pen

Continuously I am enchanted by your wisdom

Tantalized by the nectar of your conviction

I believe in you like religion

Cause you were made by God's conditions

I dream of rubbing you down with baby oil and putting you in new positions

Continuous cerebral conversations

Combined with pulsating vibrations

I dream of you in the daytime

V. E. Swanigan

Think of you in the nighttime

Cause being one with you is always the right time

I just want to remind you of my womanhood

Cause sometimes it can be forgotten and misunderstood

I am meek, humble, passionate and a sensational lover

Meaning I will sense your needs above any other

I would marry your flaws and love even your scars

You make me hit high notes in less than 10 bars

I am tired of loving you from afar

I want to be up close and personal

Not just dancing with you in my mental

Contemplating releasing myself to you

But so afraid of what you might do

If given a chance at chapter number two

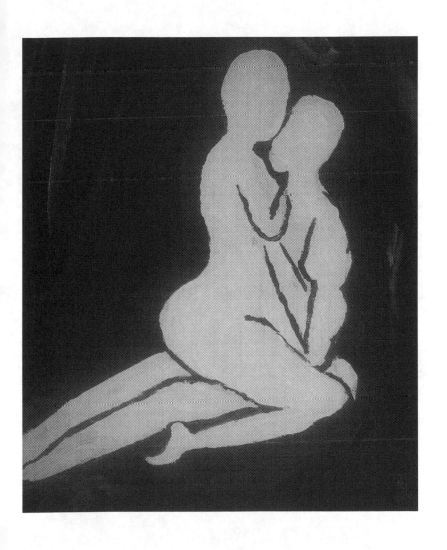

Make Love To The Page

With you I am exceptionally inspired

You set a blazing flame of desire

Your eyes pierced into the depths of my soul

And your touch ran warmth up from my toe to my elbow

I can taste your words and find nourishment in our conversation

Being with you is a fantastic cerebral ejaculation

I fantasize of the power you have over me

You give direction with good will and it amounts to ecstasy

I see the God in you and you give me love even in silence

A gentle touch from a strong hand born in resilience

A father through nature and even to other children who are down

You have been blessed to wear my king's crown

You are royalty to me a mentality of honor

I stand by you patiently as a heart donor

Because I give you all of me even in my solitude

Not disrespecting love cause as a lady I am not rude

Please I hope you understand my attitude

We are to each other a channel of directed light

V. E. Swanigan

We beam into each other's eyes a glare so bright

A love like this can't be wrong so I'll call you Mr. Right

I long for you

I could write a song for you

But hopefully this poem will do

Just to simply say this love is true

Love, Don't Go

Laying in your arms

A place so safe and warm

I feel your heart beat

Love, please don't cheat

Allow me to enjoy every second in time

Because the pleasures of you are always on my mind

Kissing your sweet lips, I smile

Wishing this will last for a while

Holding onto the scent of your cologne

Don't go to work, Love, please stay at home

I miss you when you are away and I don't want to be alone

I desire to touch your body not just to listen to you on the phone

Although our telephone conversations

Are my mental escalations

Because when I hear your voice

My soul must rejoice

V. E. Swanigan

I loved you

Without seeing you

Without touching you

Just adoring you

So love no matter what you do

Please don't go

Because my love would die without you

My love is you

Filled By An Absent Love

I hear your heartbeat even when I am away

You're close to me even when I can't stay

I see the parts of you that others can't see

Keep the lights on cause you are beautiful to me

I get turned on just from the whisper of your name

My love for you grows it feels no shame

I want to touch the inside of your soul

I want to know how it feels to spoil you

I want to take a journey with your mind

Mend all the neglected spots I can find

I smell your essence floating in the air

Even when you are not close or near

I long to kiss your lips and run my fingertips down your spine

With you, I want to spend seconds, minutes, infinities traveling through time

I want to wrap my arms around you and never let go

I want to make love to you fast and slow

I want us to be adventurous

Even to the point it's feverous

Melting and dissolving ice built shells

Tearing down to rubble protective walls

So I can melt and mold into you

V. E. Swanigan

And we build this love a new

Baby, there is just so many things I want to do

Sitting back thinking of how I could imagine us two

Intertwined, your toes touch mine

Massaging your bald head as you trace my spine

Oh with you life feels like everything is fine

I know I am your missing rib; the key to your soul, a helpmate

Together a masterpiece only God could contemplate

A nuclear explosion could flip over the planet and nothing arise

Because it would not move me more than the look in your eyes

From Your confidence even my heart expands

Your brilliance magnifies even my mind spans

I can't contain the pleasure you provide

You got my spirit open wide

Tantalized by the looks in your eyes

I bow down to you; your grace tells no lies

And I am sure to you I come as a surprise

But take me as a gift

Cause only your heart I aim to lift

Like the doctor's oath, unto you I shall do no harm

Cause I desire to keep you healthy and filled with charm

I want to keep your heart safe tenderly and warm

Your foundation, your rock, your boulder

I will be your strongest shoulder

V. E. Swanigan   20

I can taste you

Embrace you

I want to lose my mind with you

Forget about space and time with you

All I want to remember is the depths you want to go

And whether you like it better fast or slow

I want the connection with you to be all that I know

I want to feel consumed by the thoughts in your dome

I want our bodies to act like memory foam

In tune with harmony

A fantasy destiny

I love everything about you

Even the crazy things you do

You are my greatest temptation

My weakness with an exclamation

I dream of the day I can be with you

I wonder if you knew; what would you do

Cause I secretly love you

V. E. Swanigan

All Over Me

I feel it in my fingertips

Running up all the way to my lips

Trickling down my spine

Damn, Love, you came right on time

I feel it in my toes

Creeping right into my soul

I taste it with every lick of my tongue

Fill up my breath into my lung

Right through my blood stream

Damn, Love, you know what I mean

My hair follicles stand up to your attention

And you create a female erection

I feel you in every step of the sole of my feet

Even in the spaces of my teeth

You trace the curves of my limb

And I feel you til I go numb

And you engulf the tremors of my heart

It's so deep I feel like a virgin where we all start

My brain feels it but can't comprehend

I feel it all over me but I can't hold it in my hand

V. E. Swanigan

Love, you overwhelm like the sun takes over the sea

You find the space that drives my energy

You drift back and forth over me

Greater than the ocean I'm lost to your destiny

How do you feel, love?

Where do you live, love?

All Over Me

My Rain, Your Sun

If you would be for me rain

I would be for you the sun

A ray of light dawning your face

As you awake kissed by the days grace

I would keep you warm from every chill

Nurturing your body with love from afar yet and still

I'd cling to your nature as if I was right there

Making you hot

Not missing one spot

I would be for you the sun

Drying your cheeks when the rain has become too much

Filling you with a radiance that you can hardly bare

But rising slowly to your excellence

And astounded by your essence

I'd bow down to your feet

As I bring you sleep

I would be your sun

There to guide you daily from the east to the west

Helping you to persevere; watching you do your best

Always on time, even when time is all you have

V. E. Swanigan

I'd be there in an instant whenever you've lost sight

I'd brighten your day when darkness is as night

And assist you to explore a new vision

If I could be your sun

I would count the days with you

The ways with you

Even after you say I do

I'll always be there for you

To turn gray skies blue

Because I love you

And for you alone

I would be the sun

Nothing Like Before

I want you to want me like no other

Those characteristics that make you think of your mother

I can be your best friend; dedicated to you like your brother

I want to set your mind a blaze to the point you don't remember another

Can I hypnotize you like you mesmerized me?

Fill you up with love starting with your belly

I want to cook for you your favorite dish

Pass it through your lips followed by a gentle kiss

Taste your nectar while you lick your lips

Fingering licking good; just grab hold of my hips

Something like a cream puff with a tasty middle

Got you hearing love songs played on a fiddle

Cause this is not ordinary something incomparable

Got you feigning for things that are incomprehensible

Scrumptiously divine got you losing track of time

I could drink you up like a shot of tequila with lime

First you lick, then you suck, and then you swallow

My waters run deep definitely not shallow

V. E. Swanigan

I can twist and turn into you

Watch the world fall down compared to you

I even will bow down to you

Four words to describe you will not do

Matter of fact the dictionary is a thousand words too short to define your

excellence

You're a King amongst a Queen and I bask in the glory of your presence

Now take your royal staff and night me

You know go all night for me

You are sailing in my stream

And I am seeing steam

I hear the rhythms of an African drum

And your de-stressing balls make me hum

Worthy to be My Mandingo Ghana King

I will wear your Noble family ring

Cause your love makes me want to sing

I am your Queeeeeeeen to be

Cause I am coming in America ready

No longer a Princess I am your steady

The dancing shall commence like a sultry tango

You have saved me like django

But I am chained to your love

You fit into me tighter than OJ's glove

Can I wrap this love all the way around your manhood?

And pray the next day please don't let me be misunderstood

Cause I just want to love you like no other

I bear the characteristics of a good mother

Will travel the world for you, a perfect lover

Render your soul to me and watch what you discover

V. E. Swanigan

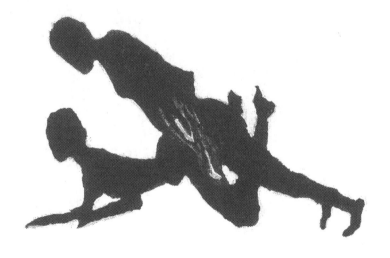

Wrapped In Your Manhood

Grasping hold of the sheets until my fingernail breaks

Filled up with your desire until my pussy leaks

One moment after the moment after my leg quakes

My rhythm with your smooth blues the bed shakes

Grinding into me deeper while holding onto feel your embrace

Sensing every sensation pulsating from your grace

I taste you on my lips even after we kiss

I feel you on my hips even when your body I miss

Just in a matter of hours we experience all of our firsts

Hoping they will be our last cause it is for you I thirst

Bending me over till I touch my toes

I even kissed you on your elbows

Cause I want to know every inch of you like a road map

So I can give you directions on how I want you to tap

You pull me over there

I kiss you on the ear

I don't care if we do it standing up or sitting in a chair

As long as you are in me, as I am into you, is all I care

Damn if you need to, Baby, you can pull back my hair

Tug on it a little; but not too tight

V. E. Swanigan

I want this to be pleasurable, oh so right

Sliding your tongue across my breast

Stimulating and ejaculating into much needed rest

Wanting to give you all of me my very best

Hoping this love will stand the test

Cause right now you are making me fly

I don't want this to end by and by

So arch my back; kiss my neck

I want you to lay out your cards; put them on the deck

I want to know how much of you I can get

Cause every time I think of you I get wet

You put me on the spot, literally

Got me feeling like a pool, not figuratively

Dripping onto you squeezing you

Drinking you up; 100 proof

You came raw; nothing but the truth

Mesmorizing My Needs

I want to memorize you to the point I make love to the lines in your smile

Pour over into your spirit and just sip your essence for a while

Stating this as a Matter of fact

I even want to memorize what you look like when I'm looking back

And I can do that for a long while

Shit, I even want to know what it looks like when your dick smile

Let me figure out the actual shape of your navel

Because X marks the spot and I am willing and able

I think the shapes of you need to be taught in preschool

So when girls turn into women looking for men they won't be made a fool

I want to glorify your body with my eyes I am so amazed

Get lost in my thoughts until I am sensually amused

Sit back and intensely watch you with my eyes closed

Not even Michelangelo could have made this

My hands and my eyes guided by your prowess

I know every dot on your body like braille

My fingers know your course they read you at will

Perusing your body until my fingers swell

I want to know you even if it hurts love

Cause as a statute of a Greek god I want to behold LOVE

V. E. Swanigan

I Remember

I am whisked away by the thoughts of you

The wind whispers your name longing for you

I would travel across oceans for you

Fly over the Seven Wonders of the World just to repeatedly soar over you

Your body is like a compass it directs my motions

Stimulates a blend of sensations like a potion

You put me through an assortment of contorted positions

Frequently I fantasize of your fantastical friction

Dripping from your lips

I recall the timber of my hips

Shaking, rattling, and rolling

Winding like a tornado uncontrolling

I can bear witness to your aptitude

It was a miraculous moment I didn't want to conclude

Now I am trapped in the memory of your presence

I remember every second redefining the word pleasure

If I could reconnect with you

Who knows what my imagination might do

But until we meet again

You shall always remain my special friend

And I shall remember

V. E. Swanigan

You Are Just Like Me

We share the same philosophy

From raising a son to making money

From staring life down to please don't judge me

When I look in your eyes I see me

We have had challenges

And made changes

We demand respect and act courageous

We give unto others and we expect the same

I'm starting to think we should share our last name

My better half that makes me whole

When in your presence I want to lose control

We smile and laugh right on cue

I am in love with me so I love what you do

Cause you brighten even my dark day

When you're around hardships don't come my way

I feel your essence, your aura, and even your chocolate skin

It is calling to me to the point I just want to jump in

All the Signs saying slow down curves ahead

But I'm still picturing your face in the morning light in our bed

Some say they don't believe in a soul mate

V. E. Swanigan

But the more I get to know you it feels like fate

Like I knew of you and you knew of me

Before we laid eyes on each other we could see

That I am perfect for you and you are perfect for me

Complications make it hard to say what will be our destiny

Facing challenges and professing truth

Wondering what will happen if we could shout it through the roof

Cause I could hear you moaning and see me screaming

Damn baby our bodies for each other is feigning

We give symbiotic a new meaning

I can see in your smile that towards me you are leaning

Getting to know you my eyes are gleaming

But I know I must wait to get that bedroom steaming

Complex timing and only God knows why

If you feel it in your soul; you will risk it to try

Cause why let something real pass you by

Not everyone will have it

Not everyone is brave enough to get it

Not everyone finds their someone

But me and you we are one

It's a matter of fact and a second of truth

You are just like me and I am just like you

Mind Fuck

Stimulate my mind; make love to my soul

Passionately stroke my ego

With cerebral masturbations

Shock my system with wise ejaculations

Penetrate my brain with the warmth of your name

Make my mouth water and my hands moisten

From your exhilarating thoughts

Exhaust me

Caress me

String me along with your words

Direct me with oral copulation

Verbal escalation

Combusting internally from an electrifying mental orgasm

MMm A mind blowing fuck

Losing Track Of Time

Brown skin on mahogany black

Whispering kisses on the curve of my back

MMMmm those caramel lips

Boy I'd like to take a sip

Cause you making my pussy drip

As we go on this tantalizing trip

Our bodies intertwined one in the same

Damn I can barely remember my own name

Your tunes; my moans; your groans

Climaxing simultaneously, giving all you own

Tempting loves sensations as they've never been known

Love is at a racing pace but don't slow down

Challenging the motion of our bodies and the flexibility of our minds

Fulfilled by your very nature every second in time

V. E. Swanigan

My Senses

You left traces of your scent on my mind and every time I think of you I forget

the essence of pain cause all my brain can recall is love

You drift in and out of my states of consciousness and I love when you play the

leading role in my dreams you're my shining knight on a white horse defining

what hero means

You confidently glide across the room as if walking on ice if you ask me I'll say

yes you don't have to ask twice

I can't defy you or deny you I am your trapped in an ivory tower princess

waiting for you to gallantly bless my lips with a long kiss

You got me drifting into places unknown feeling like I am flying when I am right

here at home

You're a taste of ecstasy when my cup is filled with a wine so bittersweet;

you're the sweet drops of honey in a gritty tea

V. E. Swanigan

You make me forget the world can be dangerous cause your love is so
courageous

You hold me close and dear even when your hands are so far from here
I still feel them perusing my soul and caressing gently in my hair

It is a glorious wonder that through space and time I am still enchanted by your
metaphysical prowess
The king of the jungle your animalistic pheromones has me overpowered like
the tigress

Your scent was expelled over my body and has been trapped in my membrane
Nothing about me since I smelled you has been the same

Cloaked in your essence and devoured by your nature
I have collapsed into the spaces of pleasure

While waiting for my deliverance unto you
I am the spectator of the creation of you

It's unexplainable that in this infinite thing we call time
All my senses still appeal to your infallible refine

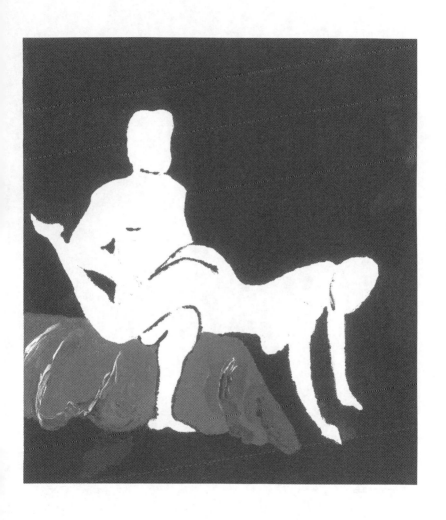

The Forbidden Fruit

Sensually sumptuous

Divinely delicious

I'd bite into you like a bee to a honeycomb

My mouth all over your body it would roam

The tantalizing taste of your nectar

The sensation of two lips coming together

I cannot just have one little taste

I'll take another bite without haste

The fragrance of your allure

Makes me desire you even more

I'd always pluck you from the tree first

With your sweet juices I'd quench my thirst

You are my mouthwatering treat

That I just can't wait to eat

Like a smorgasbord every ingredient is very versatile

Could you nourish my mind, body, and soul for a while?

Feed me, for every nibble and drop I'd devour

Like the sun feeds the land after a morning shower

V. E. Swanigan

I would not gorge you

But I would hoard you

I'm a choosey lover I know my type

So I would keep you until you were oh so ripe

Gently I'd pull back the layers to your skin

Simply cherishing my fruit; this could not be a sin

Because Of You I Am

You take my breath away

You breathe me in and I exhale your love

You climb into my soul and I'm flying like a dove

You get lost in my eyes and I can't find my way home

You cling to my breast and I'm buzzing like your ring tone

You caressed my body and it felt like it would combust

You desired my body yet conquered my mind and I knew this wasn't just lust

You were sick as a dog but I, you gave health

I am connected to you on a path since birth; you learned that to me family is wealth

I am breathing you in, and you are consumed

I am open to your declaration, and you think its four days too soon

I am breaking all boundaries and redefining the rules, and you're wondering is this feeling even cool

I am letting you know it is safe to fall; you are thinking is all this true

I am saying definitively I will catch you

Because I AM ALL READY HERE

You are acknowledging God because His love is everywhere

V. E. Swanigan

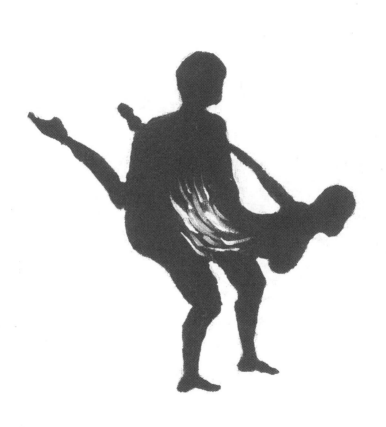

You Got Me

You got me hypnotized

With the power of your eyes

You got me trying to get to know

The magic you possess in the way you flow

You got me dreaming

Of the way we could get the bedroom steaming

You got me on the move

Trying to get close enough to show and prove

You got me hung over

My body limp and weak and it isn't any wonder

You got me

Ode To My Man

My love for you flows from my soul

And it grows deep like the roots of a tree.

Even though we don't have all that we want.

Even though we don't spend a lot of quality time together

Even though we are not who we want to be

I love the fact that we're together

It's not just your face or your warm embrace

It's not those intense eyes or that dreamy smile

It's not your witty intellect or your extreme courage

It's not just the way you walk through the fire

And always manage to put out the flame

That gives me this extra thump in my heart

That makes me cling to your name

It is the magic wand you wave over my existence

When you appear in my door way

It's the way we come together in tune

Like a musical that builds up this explosion throughout my body

This explosion of love, life, and liberty

V. E. Swanigan

You are my here and now

My tomorrow and my yesterday

You are all of me

Because you've invaded my domain

You are my everything

My Man; My Husband; My King

Answer My Prayers

The grass is always greener

When I look into your eyes

And it comes as no surprise

The way you make my temperature rise

With just one touch

I know I LOVE YOU so much

With just one laugh

I forgot about the past

You are all my dreams come true

My fantasies alive

You make me want to strive

To do what HE needs me to

It's because of you

I feel much greater

And beside you shall not falter

If only you come by me

Forever this destiny shall be

V. E. Swanigan

The If's Of Time

If I could turn back the hands of time

I would be yours and you would be mine

Heaven would be my final destination

And together we would build a nation

If I could do it all over again

I would do what it takes to make you my man

And words would flow

As emotions grow

Depicting externally

What is developing internally?

A heart felt love that will last an eternity

If I had just one more chance

To look into your eyes, it wouldn't take a second glance

For you to have me hypnotized with the essence of you

For the existence of you

Is what I desire

Combustion of love kindling a fire

You have a magnetic magnitude with a positive force

V. E. Swanigan

And I am being pulled directly to the source

Attempting to manipulate love to friendship but resistance is futile

Since your playful caring nature has me acting juvenile

If I had just one wish

It would be for a kiss

That last throughout time,

That I could do over and over again

And then press rewind

That would give me the chance

To stand face to face

And feel your warm embrace

To spend the rest of my days dawned by your grace

And to feel the enchantment of you standing in your proper place

Only if . . .

Take The Time

Allow nature to run its course

The joy from our souls will be the source

Because I am your woman in red

And thoughts of you run through my head

You have touched my soul

And with you I allow myself to let go

I am your sublime nuisance

You're a drug addicting hallucinogen

An extra heart beat before you take your last breathe

You are a misty sky that lays me to rest

So let's walk this road step by step

Smell every rose and listen to the bird's chirp

Allow life to follow the glow

Of a cherubs halo

There is no need to reconcile our differences

Because it is our flaws that stimulate our existence

Do not challenge fate

Just be patient and wait

Enjoy time and remember every second of romance

It is not given that you will get a second chance

V. E. Swanigan

Life is a constant battle

But this love don't allow it to rattle

Take a minute from your day

Just so nothing will be standing in your way

Open your eyes to the sun

Before you're trapped in a situation and wish to run

Just follow the course of events

Discovering the possibilities of passionate love heaven sent

Deep

I want you to get as much as you can stand

I want to feel you so deep you become my man

No pressure; no pain; just pleasure; no plans

Just touch me with your sensually strong hands

I want you to go so deep we become one

You below sea level moving so slow I feel you in my lung

We so far into this we the rhythm of a song unsung

I want you to go so deep from the inside I taste your cum

Hold on tight don't move let it simmer while I hum

Oh its marinating robust like a fine wine, yum

Please don't stop; but just freeze this rhythm, don't move

I want to ride out this beat, linger in the depths of your groove

So far in my nails dig into the sheets like claws

So far in you see all my scars and flaws

In so deep the words I love you dribble out my mouth

Sucking up the essence of each other, deep south

Lost in the presence of our souls you don't know where you are

Feeling like we disappeared, kidnapped to a sensual place afar

Whisk me away to the Alabama bayou

So we so deep no one can find you

Somewhere the phones don't work and computers malfunction

V. E. Swanigan

And the only Apples grow on trees not interrupting this conjunction

I want to taste only your forbidden fruit have it ripen in my mouth

Please give me more of you; peel back your layers until I see your truth

Look in the mirror and see our shimmering glory

Bodies glistening connected so tightly they telling the same story

Feeling lethargic and slightly dizzy

Legs are shaking I feel a bit woozy

Resting you inside of me and me dripping all over you

God knows what he puts together becomes one not two

Something spiritual about this combination

Like together we could build a nation

Something almost voodoo charmed and hexed

And I don't think it's just the powers of passion filled sex

I want you to want me because I will give you more than you can stand

It will be a testament to your manhood if you can handle being my man

That was only round three can you handle the rest

I want to give you all of me treat you to my very best

I need to hear your adjectives; get a full description

I want to go blow for blow with you head in a common direction

Immense ecstasy a mind, body, and soul connection

Relaxing in each other's skin

Washing away painful sin

I see you smiling will you let me in

I want to go deep then start again